How To Stop Anxiety Disorder And Panic Attacks

333 Great Tips To Control And Overcome Anxiety Attacks

ADAM COLTON

Published by BizMove
www.bizmove.com

ISBN: 1978366183
ISBN- 978-1978366183

Table of Contents

1. Anxiety Attacks Fact Sheet

Occasional anxiety is a normal part of life. You might feel anxious when faced with a problem at work, before taking a test, or making an important decision. But anxiety disorders involve more than temporary worry or fear. For a person with an anxiety disorder, the anxiety does not go away and can get worse over time. The feelings can interfere with daily activities such as job performance, school work, and relationships. There are several different types of anxiety disorders. Examples include generalized anxiety disorder, panic disorder, and social anxiety disorder.

Signs and Symptoms

Generalized Anxiety Disorder

People with generalized anxiety disorder display excessive anxiety or worry for months and face several anxiety-related symptoms.

Generalized anxiety disorder symptoms include:

- Restlessness or feeling wound-up or on edge
- Being easily fatigued

- Difficulty concentrating or having their minds go blank
- Irritability
- Muscle tension
- Difficulty controlling the worry
- Sleep problems (difficulty falling or staying asleep or restless, unsatisfying sleep)

Panic Disorder

People with panic disorder have recurrent unexpected panic attacks, which are sudden periods of intense fear that may include palpitations, pounding heart, or accelerated heart rate; sweating; trembling or shaking; sensations of shortness of breath, smothering, or choking; and feeling of impending doom.

Panic disorder symptoms include:

- Sudden and repeated attacks of intense fear
- Feelings of being out of control during a panic attack
- Intense worries about when the next attack will happen
- Fear or avoidance of places where panic attacks have occurred in the past

Social Anxiety Disorder

People with social anxiety disorder (sometimes called "social phobia") have a marked fear of social or performance situations in which they expect to feel embarrassed, judged, rejected, or fearful of offending others.

Social anxiety disorder symptoms include:

- Feeling highly anxious about being with other people and having a hard time talking to them
- Feeling very self-conscious in front of other people and worried about feeling humiliated, embarrassed, or rejected, or fearful of offending others
- Being very afraid that other people will judge them
- Worrying for days or weeks before an event where other people will be
- Staying away from places where there are other people
- Having a hard time making friends and keeping friends
- Blushing, sweating, or trembling around other people
- Feeling nauseous or sick to your stomach when other people are around

Evaluation for an anxiety disorder often begins with a visit to a primary care provider. Some physical health conditions, such as an overactive thyroid or low blood sugar, as well as taking certain medications, can imitate or worsen an anxiety disorder. A thorough mental health evaluation is also helpful, because anxiety disorders often co-exist with other related conditions, such as depression or obsessive-compulsive disorder.

Risk Factors

Researchers are finding that genetic and environmental factors, frequently in interaction with one another, are risk factors for anxiety disorders. Specific factors include:

- Shyness, or behavioral inhibition, in childhood
- Being female
- Having few economic resources
- Being divorced or widowed
- Exposure to stressful life events in childhood and adulthood
- Anxiety disorders in close biological relatives
- Parental history of mental disorders
- Elevated afternoon cortisol levels in the saliva (specifically for social anxiety disorder)

Treatments and Therapies

Anxiety disorders are generally treated with psychotherapy, medication, or both.

Psychotherapy

Psychotherapy or "talk therapy" can help people with anxiety disorders. To be effective, psychotherapy must be directed at the person's specific anxieties and tailored to his or her needs. A typical "side effect" of psychotherapy is temporary discomfort involved with thinking about confronting feared situations.

Cognitive Behavioral Therapy (CBT)

CBT is a type of psychotherapy that can help people with anxiety disorders. It teaches a person different ways of thinking, behaving, and reacting to anxiety-producing and fearful situations. CBT can also help people learn and practice social skills, which is vital for treating social anxiety disorder.

Two specific stand-alone components of CBT used to treat social anxiety disorder are **cognitive therapy** and **exposure therapy**. Cognitive therapy focuses on identifying, challenging, and then neutralizing unhelpful thoughts underlying anxiety disorders.

Exposure therapy focuses on confronting the fears underlying an anxiety disorder in order to help people engage in activities they have been avoiding. Exposure therapy is used along with relaxation exercises and/or imagery. One study, called a meta-analysis because it pulls together all of the previous studies and calculates the statistical magnitude of the combined effects, found that cognitive therapy was superior to exposure therapy for treating social anxiety disorder.

CBT may be conducted individually or with a group of people who have similar problems. Group therapy is particularly effective for social anxiety disorder. Often "homework" is assigned for participants to complete between sessions.

Self-Help or Support Groups

Some people with anxiety disorders might benefit from joining a self-help or support group and sharing their problems and achievements with others. Internet chat rooms might also be useful, but any advice received over the Internet should be used with caution, as Internet acquaintances have usually never seen each other and false identities are common. Talking with a trusted friend or member of the clergy can also provide support, but it is not necessarily a sufficient alternative to care from an expert clinician.

Stress-Management Techniques

Stress management techniques and meditation can help people with anxiety disorders calm themselves and may enhance the effects of therapy. While there is evidence that aerobic exercise has a calming effect, the quality of the studies is not strong enough to support its use as treatment. Since caffeine, certain illicit drugs, and even some over-the-counter cold medications can aggravate the symptoms of anxiety disorders, avoiding them should be considered. Check with your physician or pharmacist before taking any additional medications.

The family can be important in the recovery of a person with an anxiety disorder. Ideally, the family should be supportive but not help perpetuate their loved one's symptoms.

Medication

Medication does not cure anxiety disorders but often relieves symptoms. Medication can only be prescribed by a medical doctor (such as a psychiatrist or a primary care provider), but a few states allow psychologists to prescribe psychiatric medications.

Medications are sometimes used as the initial treatment of an anxiety disorder, or are used only if there is insufficient response to a course of psychotherapy. In research studies, it is common for patients treated with a combination of psychotherapy and medication to have better outcomes than those treated with only one or the other.

The most common classes of medications used to combat anxiety disorders are antidepressants, anti-anxiety drugs, and beta-blockers. Be aware that some medications are effective only if they are taken regularly and that symptoms may recur if the medication is stopped.

Antidepressants

Antidepressants are used to treat depression, but they also are helpful for treating anxiety disorders. They take several weeks to start working and may cause side effects such as headache, nausea, or difficulty sleeping. The side effects are usually not a problem for most people, especially if the dose starts off low and is increased slowly over time.

Please Note: Although antidepressants are safe and effective for many people, they may be risky for children, teens, and young adults. A "black box" warning—the most serious type of warning that a prescription can carry—has been added to the labels of antidepressants. The labels now warn that antidepressants may cause some people to have suicidal thoughts or make suicide attempts. For this reason, anyone taking an antidepressant should be monitored closely, especially when they first start taking the medication.

Anti-Anxiety Medications

Anti-anxiety medications help reduce the symptoms of anxiety, panic attacks, or extreme fear and worry. The most common anti-anxiety medications are called benzodiazepines. Benzodiazepines are first-line treatments for generalized anxiety disorder. With panic disorder or social phobia (social anxiety disorder), benzodiazepines are usually second-line treatments, behind antidepressants.

Beta-Blockers

Beta-blockers, such as propranolol and atenolol, are also helpful in the treatment of the physical symptoms of anxiety, especially social anxiety. Physicians prescribe them to control rapid heartbeat, shaking, trembling, and blushing in anxious situations.

Choosing the right medication, medication dose, and treatment plan should be based on a person's needs and medical situation, and done under an expert's care. Only an expert clinician can help you decide whether the medication's ability to help is worth the risk of a side effect. Your doctor may try several medicines before finding the right one.

You and your doctor should discuss:

- How well medications are working or might work to improve your symptoms
- Benefits and side effects of each medication
- Risk for serious side effects based on your medical history
- The likelihood of the medications requiring lifestyle changes
- Costs of each medication
- Other alternative therapies, medications, vitamins, and supplements you are taking and how these may affect your treatment
- How the medication should be stopped. Some drugs can't be stopped abruptly but must be tapered off slowly under a doctor's supervision.

2. 333 Great Tips To Control And Overcome Anxiety Attacks

Anxiety is a medical issue faced by people of all ages and races. If you allow it to control your life, it will. Using this advice, you can see options that may help you with your anxiety.

1. Deal with your daily stress to manage your anxiety. When stress levels increase, anxiety levels also tend to increase. One important skill to learn is delegation. Take some time to relax and do things you enjoy everyday.

2. Listening to music is a great way to deal with anxiety. Try putting on some music you enjoy the next time you find yourself in the throes of an anxiety attack. Follow each note and get lost in the music. Soon, your mind will forget about what is causing you anxiety. Keeping your brain busy can really help deal with anxiety.

3. If you are suffering from frequent bouts of anxiety, it will help you to confide in another person, rather than to keep it inside. Bottling up anxiety only makes it worse, while talking about

it with another person can diffuse the bomb and allow you go get some support!

4. Starting a gratitude journal can go a long way in helping you cope with your anxiety. Write down things you are thankful for each day, and elaborate as much as you can. This gives you things to refer back to when you are dealing with your anxiety. A journal can really help you focus on what is most important during these times.

5. Learn more about anxiety, and how it may be affecting you personally. Just having terms to describe your condition can really help you feel better and may be all the motivation you need to face and fight the fear. Anxiety is too debilitating a condition to take lying down, so educate you to further action.

6. Work on having good posture. Having bad posture compresses organs, cuts off circulation and shortens breathing. Many times, it is easy, even under a normal amount of anxiety, to sit in positions that cause harm to our body. Try not to do this, as this will better your health and help decrease the amount of anxiety you endure.

7. Give yourself daily goals, and strive to achieve it. Doing this will give you something to focus on

each day, which helps to eliminate those negative and anxious feelings you may have. You should think about constructive things and not negatives.

8. Make time for practicing some relaxation techniques. There are various techniques that you can work into your schedule too. Relaxation techniques like progressive muscle relaxation, mindfulness meditation, and some deep breathing may reduce your anxiety symptoms, and help you feel more relaxed so you can have a better emotional well-being.

9. It is always a good idea to talk about your problems when the need arises. The only exception to this is, when you are having an anxiety attack. This can be absolutely devastating to your chances of coming out of the anxiety attack in a healthy manner. Make sure you remain positive during any anxiety attacks.

10. Reduce your level of anxiety by asking others for help when you need it. Many people feel that asking for help is a sign of weakness, but it is actually a very intelligent thing to do when a task is more than you can handle. Delegating appropriate tasks to others will keep anxiety under control.

11. Do not approach life or problems as a black-or-white situation. The world is awash with shades of grey. When you realize that the worst-case scenario is not the only outcome for a problem, you can understand that you have options to solve the issue. Control your thinking by not dealing in absolutes.

12. Don't be afraid to talk to others about what you are feeling. Holding these fears inside is only going to make your situation worse. Instead, find a friend or family member who you trust or even, a registered counselor to talk to. Just a few minutes a week of good venting can do wonders for how you manage and feel.

13. When excessive worry, and anxiety takes control of your mind, stop, and write down the things that are bothering you. Putting your worries in writing, allows you to see, and evaluate the source of your anxiety. Take action on the things that you can resolve. Release the items that are beyond your control.

14. Watch what triggers your anxiety, and name them. This can help you better understand your triggers so that you can be conscious of your decisions when you have to deal with them.

15. Start writing in a gratitude journal. At the end of each day, write down at least five things you were grateful for. Become aware of all the wonderful positive things in your life and shift your focus away from dwelling on things that trigger worry, stress or negativity.

16. Anxiety can take a lot out of you, both emotionally and physically. On top of seeing a physician, you should have an organized plan in place. Without organization, dealing with your anxiety will become sporadic and unhealthy. You must be organized when coping and dealing with your anxiety attacks.

17. While it can be beneficial to have low anxiety, high anxiety is a problem. You should learn to tell the difference between the kind of anxiety that motivates you to try harder, and stress that is crippling and makes you want to give up.

18. Stop being a victim of your mind. You are the primary controller of your feelings and thoughts. While this may seem common knowledge, humans are always forgetting to take control of their mind, and instead, let it control them. You are the driving force in your mental approach

and attitude towards problems. Create a positive way of handling situations.

19. In order to make sure you are not overwhelmed by anxiety, exercise often. Endorphins, which are produced from physical activity, will keep your mind off of your stress and relax you. Physical activity is also recommended for general health.

20. Take control of your emotions. The way you feel can often cause anxiety. Once you have the discipline to control your emotions, you can rid yourself of anxiety. You may have to learn to emotionally detach yourself from feelings to gain control of your emotions and eliminate anxiety for good.

21. Positive interaction is a must when you are going through rough anxiety. Helping others is a great cure for anxiety. Find a neighbor or a friend who needs a helping hand, and watch it work wonders for how you feel. There is no better medicine than helping other people in times of need.

22. One of the ways that you can feel better during the day and help reduce anxiety is to stretch the moment that you wake up. This can help limit any strain on your body when you go to work or

school and can help generate the relaxation of all your muscles.

23. If anxiety has got you feeling you down, one way to help lessen your angst is to exercise. When you exercise, it releases positive endorphins in the brain which have you feeling better. Not only will you feel more positive, and decrease the stress that is causing your anxiety, you will get in good shape, too!

24. Come up with daily objectives. By having a daily goal, you can set your focus on that rather than anxiety. Keeping yourself busy will help you prevent anxiety attacks.

25. Talk to a trusted friend or family member about your anxiety problems. If you tell someone else how you feel, they may be able to help you put things in perspective and help you to think positive thoughts. This can help you get rid of anxiety or at least make it better.

26. If you suffer from anxiety, try your best to quit smoking, as soon as possible. Smoking reduces the functionality of many different organs in your body, putting you in a position where you may be more stressed than usual. Quitting

smoking can refresh your body and increase your overall outlook on life.

27. When you are suffering from high anxiety and stress, your body may keep you awake, at times, and cause insomnia. There are a number of natural sleep aids on the market that can help you sleep, or you can go to the doctor and try using a prescription that can help you get the sleep your body needs.

28. Try to have a thicker skin when you are dealing with your emotions. If you have strong feelings about something, you are more likely to feel negative about something and worry, which leads to serious anxiety issues. Practice some emotional detachment when you are going through your everyday proceedings.

29. If you want to manage your anxiety, it's crucial that you get all the sleep you need. Sleep deprivation, which can cause mental and physical problems, is a major factor in the cause of anxiety. Adult should get seven to eight hours of sleep every night.

30. Give yourself a goal to reach for every day, and try your best to attain it. Doing this will give you something to focus on each day, which helps to

eliminate those negative and anxious feelings you may have. Instead, focus on constructive thoughts.

31. The best way to deal with anxiety is to learn how to minimize it. Many people do this through deep breathing methods. This is a great way to learn how to control your own emotions and bring a level of balance into your life, while improving your mind.

32. Always keep your promises to yourself, as well as, to others. Anxiety can come on from feelings of inadequacy because you make promises to yourself or others that you fear you cannot live up to. If you promise yourself a vacation, for instance, do not let fear and doubt about going, cause you to break another promise to yourself. This will only lead to more anxiety.

33. Take more Vitamin C. Did you know that humans are the only ones that can not make their own Vitamin C? In contrast, when many animals are under stress, their bodies produce large quantities of Vitamin C. So, if you are under a lot of stress or experiencing high anxiety, take a supplement that is high in Vitamin C to help.

34. Get more than one medical opinion. Different doctors treat different conditions differently. One doctor may prescribe anxiety medicine, while another might only recommend therapy. Get more than one opinion about what you can do so that you can conquer your anxiety, and make sure you understand all the options available to you.

35. If you discover that watching television causes your anxiety levels to go up, then turn it off. Limit the amount of time that you watch television, and do something more productive instead. Try cleaning the house, exercising, hanging out with friends, or reading a good book. Television time should be limited. Never watch anything that causes you to stress out immediately upon watching.

36. Give it time. Sometimes the healing process from anxiety related issues can be very gradual. Many times you might not feel like you are making any progress at all. The key to this is to understand that it takes time. When you look back over the months you will notice your progress, and after a year, you will be able to notice a significant change.

37. Proper breathing is essential to reducing sudden feelings of anxiety. Using a count to control your breathing can be an effective way to reduce anxious feelings. Pick a count, such as 3 in, and 3 out. Repeat this pattern, until the feelings of anxiety have resolved, and passed.

38. A good way to get rid of your anxiety is to treat yourself to a snack that you like. When you start to feel a bit anxious, one of the best ways to calm yourself, is to make your taste buds happy. When you make your taste buds happy, your stomach is happy, and then you're happy.

39. Starting a gratitude journal can go a long way in helping you cope with your anxiety. Write down things you are thankful for each day, and elaborate as much as you can. This gives you things to refer back to when you are dealing with your anxiety. A journal can really help you focus on what is most important during these times.

40. Talk to a trusted friend or family member about your anxiety problems. If you tell someone else how you feel, they may be able to help you put things in perspective and help you to think positive thoughts. This can help you get rid of anxiety or at least make it better.

41. Therapy, in conjunction with keeping a journal, can really help you when dealing with your anxiety. It can help you realize what the anxiety is stemming from and you can then talk to your therapist about it. Talking to others and discussing your problems is always a good idea.

42. If you believe you are suffering from symptoms related to anxiety disorder, the very first person that you should discuss this issue with is your primary care physician. Your family doctor will be able to inform you whether the symptoms that are causing you alarm are caused by an anxiety disorder, another medical problem, or a combination of the two.

43. Exercise is one of the best things that you can do to help eliminate any anxiety that you feel. When you exercise, your body flushes out all of the toxins from the inside out, which can improve your body functionality. Exercise at least one hour per day to improve the way that you feel.

44. You must realize that anxiety is your mind telling you that you need something. Whether it is something simple like a break, or just the need to talk to a friend or family member, you should address the cause. If your anxiety is creeping up

because you need to handle something; handle it. You will thank yourself later.

45. Do not drink alcohol or consume nicotine in any form if at all possible. A lot of people think that these things will relax you, but ultimately they don't. They can even make your anxiety worse. Look to healthier methods including relaxation exercises, fun social interaction and sound dietary habits.

46. Exercise. Get into doing some sort of daily exercise routine. Go for a walk or a run, join the gym, or buy a workout DVD that you do each day. This extra activity releases dopamine and seratonin into your body, boosts your mood and your oxygen levels. All of these things work together to keep you healthier, happier and less stressed.

47. A great way to help you deal with your anxiety is to identify the things that bring it on. When you determine what causes your anxiety, you can better prepare yourself to deal with those situations should they arise in the future. This way, you can see what specific things you need to work on.

48. If you have a problem trying to relax, in order to release all of your anxiety, you should consider aromatherapy. There are several herbs and flowers that can ease moods, once the aromas are inhaled. Essential oils containing peppermint, bay, anise, and thyme, are a few examples of the scents that you may find effective.

49. Immediately respond if you are having an anxiety attack at night while you are trying to sleep. Getting out of bed is vital; it can be helpful to drink some water, have a snack, or watch a little television, too. Keep yourself in motion though, as this will get rid of the anxiety attack faster, allowing you to return to your rest.

50. Whenever you are feeling high anxiety, try to take deep breaths. Take these breaths from your stomach and hold it in for a few seconds before releasing it. It is recommended that you do this 5 to 8 times. This can really help relax you, and make your anxiety disappear.

51. Perhaps the most important step with dealing with anxiety is admitting that you have a problem. Once you admit to yourself that you have an issue with anxiety, you can put yourself in a mindset where you are prepared to deal with

it. Admitting you have a problem is the first step to recovery.

52. If your anxiety level is at an all time high you can help your mood by engaging in some type of healthy sexual activity. When people have sex it releases endorphins into the blood, which will send signals to the brain that it needs to be in a much better mood.

53. Some great supplements to take if you are experiencing anxiety are cod liver, krill or fish oil. There have been studies that have shown that these three oils are as effective as many of the prescription medications that are available on the market for treating anxiety and depression. A good rule of thumb is 1,000 to 2,000 mg, per day.

54. Breathe easy. When you start to feel anxious, try to concentrate on breathing correctly. Inhale through your nostrils for about two seconds, and then exhale through parted lips for four seconds. Continue this routine for a full minute. Once your breathing gets back to normal, follow it up with a couple of minutes of soothing, positive self-talk.

55. Think happy thoughts. If you have problems falling asleep at night because of anxiety, think about everything good in your life and the positive things you are going to do the next day. While it may seem hard to do at first, the more you do it, the more you will get used to it.

56. Learn how to use positive affirmations to help you with your anxiety. This can include motivational poetry, upbeat songs or just simple phrases that make you feel good about yourself. Sit down and think about how you want your day to go and do what you have to do to make it a reality.

57. When dealing with increased anxiety, you will probably have an increased desire for salt. This happens because your body actually needs salt and is asking you to consume it. Unprocessed raw salt is the optimum variant to use, since your body can digest it easiest and get trace minerals from it.

58. If your anxiety is so bad that you have a hard time sleeping you should adjust your nightly ritual accordingly. Avoid watching things like horror films and action movies that creates negative feelings that persist once you go to bed.

Try watching more relaxing programming or listening to music before you head to bed.

59. Help others whenever you have a chance. If you see someone that needs help, ask them. You may also find an opportunity to help out family and friends by simply asking them if they need anything. This will keep your mind off of anxiety and will help you feel better about yourself.

60. Reduce the anxiety in your life by learning to say no to situations that cause you stress. There is no reason to feel that you must be available to fulfill every request that is asked of you. Learn not to accept responsibility for more than you are able to handle comfortably.

61. No matter who you find, seek assistance to discuss your problems. Support systems make dealing with anxiety easier. Talking about anxiety not only helps you to better understand it but also to control it.

62. It is always a good idea to talk about your problems when the need arises. The only exception to this is, when you are having an anxiety attack. This can be absolutely devastating to your chances of coming out of the anxiety

attack in a healthy manner. Make sure you remain positive during any anxiety attacks.

63. Find some reasons to laugh at the world. You can watch a funny movie or television show and this will also take your mind off of any worries you might have to deal with. So find a comedy on the television, sit back, and do not forget to let out those laughs.

64. You should respond immediately if you have anxiety attacks at night while sleeping. It's helpful to get up and move around, eat a light snack, watch tv or get a drink of water. Keep yourself in motion though, as this will get rid of the anxiety attack faster, allowing you to return to your rest.

65. Exercise often. Working out, regardless of what activity you choose to engage in, will help you feel less anxious. Studies have shown that aerobic activities can help people as much as some kinds of medication. They are able to alter the way the brain works, even protecting it to a certain extent.

66. Anxiety, like so many other things, is neither good or bad. The real problem is when anxiety begins to have other impacts on your life. If you feel as though your anxiety is reaching dangerous

levels, then you know it is time to talk to a medical professional about your options.

67. Taking alcohol out of the picture. Alcohol is a depressant and can severely impact your approach to issues. When you drink, your mind is clouded and you can easily begin to obsess over issues. Minimize your drinking and the amounts you imbibe when you do. Keeping a clear head makes for clear thoughts.

68. Relaxation is not so easy during times of an anxiety attack. However, relaxation, prayer and meditation, can really help reduce anxiety by making a habit of these activities in your daily life. This helps nurture your spirit and relax your physical body, the way it needs to be relaxed, instead of sitting there inactive, watching television.

69. Find and address the causes of your stress and anxiety. If financial fears are keeping you up at night, talk to a debt counselor or financial advisor and start setting up a budget. If you have fears about your health, make an appointment with your doctor for a physical. Taking action and being proactive can help you face your fears and address them head-on, before they spiral out of control.

70. Get a pet. If you are experiencing worry and anxiety try getting a pet. Taking care of your pet and going for walks with him or her can help you deal with anxiety. It also provides you with a friend that you can spend your time with instead of worrying.

71. Learn how to distract yourself. As soon as you feel the anxiety starting to overwhelm you, find something that offers a distraction. Make sure that it's something that takes up a lot of concentration or energy, such as a difficult puzzle or a brisk workout. By concentrating on something other than your anxiety, you will find that it disappears quite quickly.

72. If you frequently suffer from bouts of anxiety that appear seemingly out of nowhere, or you feel anxious a majority of the time, you may have what is called generalized anxiety disorder. This disorder needs to be treated by an experienced doctor, or therapist before anxiety has a chance to take over your life.

73. If you have an anxiety disorder, it may be wise to seek out a support group for people with anxiety disorder and panic attack. Being around others who share your symptoms can be a great

comfort and will allow you to share ideas for controlling anxiety and overcoming your fears.

74. One of the ways that you can feel better during the day and help reduce anxiety is to stretch the moment that you wake up. This can help limit any strain on your body when you go to work or school and can help generate the relaxation of all your muscles.

75. Remember to keep the good parts of your life in mind. List some of the positives in your life upn rising and also right before bed. The upbeat thoughts can prevent negative ones from entering your mind and help prevent negative feelings which fuel your anxiety.

76. Keep yourself as busy as you possibly can. Being very active helps prevent any anxiety that may occur. As soon as you get up in the mornings, begin doing something immediately. Make sure you keep yourself busy all day long. Clean up the house, walk the dog, clean up your garden, read, or exercise. All these things can decrease your anxiety. Remaining idle just causes you to think about the negative things that are occurring in your life, which makes your anxiety worse.

77. If you suffer from anxiety, try your best to quit smoking, as soon as possible. Smoking reduces the functionality of many different organs in your body, putting you in a position where you may be more stressed than usual. Quitting smoking can refresh your body and increase your overall outlook on life.

78. Did you know that it is almost impossible to suffer from depression and anxiety when you are laughing? Laughter is great medicine for fighting anxiety. There has been a lot of research on the subject, but it does not take a scientist to know that when you are laughing, you are not depressed.

79. A great way to help you deal with your anxiety is to identify the things that bring it on. When you determine what causes your anxiety, you can better prepare yourself to deal with those situations should they arise in the future. This way, you can see what specific things you need to work on.

80. If you feel like nothing is working for your anxiety and your doctor recommends it, take medication. Many people do not like the idea of relying on medication for assistance, but sometimes, it is the only thing that works. But,

only resort to this if your doctor feels it is needed.

81. Limit caffeine and other stimulants. Too much caffeine in a healthy person's diet can induce feelings of anxiety, so in someone who is already struggling with this disorder, it can have disastrous effects. Caffeine and other stimulants enhance alertness by blocking certain chemicals in the brain, and in individuals predisposed to anxiety, can cause increased heart rate, sweating palms, ringing in the ears, and even panic attacks.

82. Make sure you are aware of your anxiety trigger points, and articulate what they are. This gives you greater control over your anxiety.

83. There is more than one type of anxiety that exists. If you are unsure of what kind of anxiety you are experiencing, you should discuss things with your doctor before trying to find medication or other sources of help. This professional will be able to help you identify your triggers.

84. Some people who have been diagnosed with anxiety disorder are prescribed medication by their mental health professional. If your physician has determined that you need

medication to aid in the treatment of your anxiety disorder, it is important that you take it as directed. Never abruptly stop taking it. If you are having some side effects from your medication, discuss these issues with your doctor. It is also important to remember that some medications will cause a bad reaction, if they are not tapered off gradually while under a doctor's care.

85. Get more than one medical opinion. Different doctors treat different conditions differently. One doctor may prescribe anxiety medicine, while another might only recommend therapy. Get more than one opinion about what you can do so that you can conquer your anxiety, and make sure you understand all the options available to you.

86. If you suffer from anxiety and can't get out that much, consider getting yourself a pet. They are shown to have numerous benefits, like lowering blood pressure and stress. The companionship an animal can offer is that they are unequivocally loyal, pleasant and will not get you all stressed out like other people can make you.

87. Separate yourself from things that cause you anxiety for a few hours every day. If you find

that thinking about something too often is making you anxious, go on a walk or somewhere you like for a while. Thinking about something too much can just make it worse, so keep your mind occupied.

88. To help you reduce your anxiety symptoms, keep a journal of all of the events or issues that make you anxious throughout the day. Refer back to these events and see how they actually transpired. You will realize that you are often imagining a worst case scenario which does not transpire.

89. Listening to music is an excellent anxiety reducer. If you feel like you are suffering from anxiety, put on your favorite album. Focus on each note in the music. After a little while, your mind will begin to relax. If you keep your mind occupied, you will find that you have less time to worry about your anxiety.

90. If you discover that your anxiety is causing you to be in a bad mood, try getting enough exercise each day in order to calm yourself. The endorphins produced by exercising help you to keep a positive attitude and take your mind away from issues that are bothersome and cause stress.

Additionally, exercise is something that should be included in your daily routine.

91. Try not to watch the news often. Many times, the news is filled with all kinds of negative stories, about occurrences in your town, and around the world. When dealing with anxiety, you do not need to feed the anxiety anymore negative issues to dwell on. Turn off the TV, pick up a lighthearted book to read instead.

92. Set daily goals. By having something to strive for each day, your mind will stay focused on something positive. Doing this keeps your mind active, and can help prevent the occurrence of negative ideas or thoughts which lead to anxiety attacks.

93. When you start feeling anxious in public, find ways to distract yourself. When in line at the store, start looking at the items hanging near you or the products in your basket. Observe the ceiling, count the number of checkstands, and do anything else you can to preoccupy your mind and keep it from dwelling on anxious thoughts.

94. You should try to add some deep breathing techniques to your daily schedule, if you are suffering from feelings of anxiety. If you breathe

from the diaphragm, it brings oxygen to your blood and that will help you to relax right away. Any time that you feel overwhelmed, you should take a minute to do this.

95. Anxieties are unavoidable, but when you are faced with a situation that makes you anxious, remember to take deep breaths. Breathe in like you are smelling a flower, and breathe out like you are trying to blow out a candle. This will give you more oxygen, slow your heartbeat and calm you down.

96. Reduce the anxiety in your life by learning to say no to situations that cause you stress. There is no reason to feel that you must be available to fulfill every request that is asked of you. Learn not to accept responsibility for more than you are able to handle comfortably.

97. Relieve your unfounded worries, by doing some research. Statistics, facts, and other pieces of information can help you feel more secure. Learning more about what is bothering you can also show you that you don't, in fact, have anything to worry about. If doing the research yourself might worsen your anxiety, ask a friend, or family member to help.

98. Begin a journal, and every day, write down at least one thing positive in your life. Then, whenever your anxiety begins to bother you, open and read your journal. This will remind you of all the good things you have in life and help keep your anxiety to a minimum.

99. Learn how to meditate. There are many different ways to meditate, and they all have the effect of releasing your mind from anxious thoughts. Meditation is not something that you ever conquer, so do not worry about doing it right. An easy way to practice meditation is to light a candle and gently gaze at the flame for 10 minutes. Sit quietly, and just let your thoughts pass through your mind without stopping them.

100.   Want an easy way to reduce feelings of anxiety? Having a positive attitude and smiling as much as possible is key. Stay conscious of the good things in your life. If you feel an anxiety attack coming on, find something funny to laugh about.

101.   If you are feeling anxious as you try to settle down for the night, take action to stop it immediately before it gets worse. Drinking or eating something, or watching a bit of your favorite TV show, can help soothe your anxious

thoughts. Be sure you're constantly moving so you're able to rid yourself of the anxiety quicker. This will allow you to return to bed and get better sleep more quickly.

102.   Don't be afraid to talk to others about what you are feeling. Holding these fears inside is only going to make your situation worse. Instead, find a friend or family member who you trust or even, a registered counselor to talk to. Just a few minutes a week of good venting can do wonders for how you manage and feel.

103.   Have a trusted resource to call on, whenever you may be subject to an attack. Be it a relative or friend, you should have someone who is aware of your condition and can help talk you through an attack. Having to face one alone is very overwhelming, and you will work through them quicker if you have someone to help.

104.   Learn how to distract yourself. As soon as you feel the anxiety starting to overwhelm you, find something that offers a distraction. Make sure that it's something that takes up a lot of concentration or energy, such as a difficult puzzle or a brisk workout. By concentrating on something other than your anxiety, you will find that it disappears quite quickly.

105.   To help manage your anxiety, consider meeting with a therapist who specializes in cognitive behavioral therapy. This kind of therapy can help you attack specific fears or worries by identifying and changing distorted patterns in your thinking. By looking at the full picture of how your worries affect you, you can hopefully decrease your overall anxiety when those thinking patterns are eliminated.

106.   If you are suffering from anxiety, one of the best things that you can do is to drink a lot of water during the day. Eight glasses of water can help to reduce the toxins in your body and put you in the best position to stay positive during the day.

107.   Positive interaction is a must when you are going through rough anxiety. Helping others is a great cure for anxiety. Find a neighbor or a friend who needs a helping hand, and watch it work wonders for how you feel. There is no better medicine than helping other people in times of need.

108.   Don't forget to play. With the hustle and bustle of your busy life, taking the time to play a sport, a game or an instrument might seem

frivolous. Taking an hour to let your hair down and have fun can do wonders for your stress and anxiety levels, though.

109.   Do not feel embarrassed or ashamed to seek professional help if your anxiety has become something that you cannot effectively deal with on your own. It will help you to talk to a doctor and let those feelings out. They will then, be able to prescribe you something that can help you, if that is what is needed.

110.   Exercise is one of the best things that you can do to help eliminate any anxiety that you feel. When you exercise, your body flushes out all of the toxins from the inside out, which can improve your body functionality. Exercise at least one hour per day to improve the way that you feel.

111.   If going to sleep is a problem, take a few minutes to write down your worries in a journal. Just a few minutes spent writing your problems down on paper can assist you in getting your thoughts out, helping you with sleep. Try writing every night or whenever you feel the need to do so.

112.   Do not fear seeking medical advice for facing your anxiety. Just the thought of seeking a professional opinion, can be another source of anxiety. Don't let this happen to you. Anxiety is often a medical condition that can be solved with the right information and treatment. Relax and make the appointment.

113.   Learn how to release anxious feelings with the help of emotional releasing techniques. Learn The Sedona Method or the Emotional Freedom Technique. These methods help you get to the root of your anxiety, and keep releasing it until you are completely relaxed. The information on these methods is either free or low-cost and can be found through a web search.

114.   Schedule a time for exploring your doubts and worries. Remind yourself not to think about these issues until it is time. Then set aside an hour to deal with any issues. It is time to stop indulging in worry once your allotted time has elapsed. Since this approach is structured, it is a great way to control your feelings.

115.   Perhaps the most important step with dealing with anxiety is admitting that you have a problem. Once you admit to yourself that you have an issue with anxiety, you can put yourself

in a mindset where you are prepared to deal with it. Admitting you have a problem is the first step to recovery.

116.	Have you ever enjoyed listening to music and singing out loud? If you suffer from an anxiety attack, try playing your absolute favorite music and singing it as loud as you can. This is very helpful, and it will put a smile on your face. Try this next time during an anxiety attack.

117.	You should consult a doctor. A lot of people who suffer from anxiety, do not think that their feelings warrant a trip to the doctor, but the truth is that there are many factors that could cause anxiety, and the doctor will be able to best diagnose the causes. Because the doctor will determine the underlying cause of your anxiety, he can properly prescribe the right solution for you.

118.	When you try and deal with anxiety try both a natural and medical approach. Your physician can look over your personal affliction and prescribe or suggest specific medications. However, on the other hand, you can see positive changes through natural methods, like changing your diet. Those who use several different kinds of treatments tend to have more success.

119.   Find a visual or aural anchor that makes you feel calm or relaxed. Try to choose something abundant and ever-present, such as clouds or water. When you feel anxious, look to the sky or play a soothing track of flowing water on an mp3 player. These anchors can give you a focal point when you feel anxious and head off a full-blown panic attack.

120.   Begin your day with a few minutes of positive affirmations. Tell yourself how you want your day to go. Make sure you are using cheerful and motivating words when applying this method. This can help your day go a lot better, which can minimize your anxiety throughout the entire day.

121.   Focus on the positives in life. Try to think about these positive things each evening and morning. Positive thinking helps keep negative thoughts from consuming you, which will help reduce the anxiety that you feel.

122.   Watch how much alcohol you drink. If you are going out with your friends to drink, then try to reduce your alcohol consumption. Alcohol

can do damage to your body while increasing the amount of stress that you have in the long-term. Also, alcohol puts you in many dangerous situations that can yield more anxiety.

123.   During times when you feel anxious, watching an enjoyable comedy can be helpful. This genre can help bring laughter to your life, offer a new perspective and take your mind off of the troubles that caused your anxiety.

124.   Try to minimize the amount of negative words that you are using or negative comments that you are making. The more negative talk you do, the more negative thoughts and anxiety that can come creeping into your head, causing you unneeded health issues that will affect your life in some very bad ways.

125.   After being diagnosed with anxiety disorder, many people worry about the cost associated with needed medical intervention. Most insurance plans will cover needed medicines and treatments for this disorder. If you currently do not have health insurance, contact your county government's Health and Human Services division. In many instances, they offer mental health care at a nearby public health facility.

Charges at these facilities are pro-rated on a person's ability to pay.

126.   An excellent way to get a handle on anxiety, is to locate the source of it. Are you feelings more stress at the workplace? If so, maybe there are steps you can take to lower your stress level, such as asking your supervisor if there is an opportunity for you to change to a different team or project. If you know the source of your anxiety, it is possible to start eradicating it.

127.   If you have a problem trying to relax, in order to release all of your anxiety, you should consider aromatherapy. There are several herbs and flowers that can ease moods, once the aromas are inhaled. Essential oils containing peppermint, bay, anise, and thyme, are a few examples of the scents that you may find effective.

128.   If your sleep gets interrupted by a serious anxiety attack, take action against it immediately. Find a distracting but relaxing activity, such as reading a book, to help distract and relax you. Keep yourself in motion though, as this will get rid of the anxiety attack faster, allowing you to return to your rest.

129.   If you suffer from anxiety, you may want to consider seeing a therapist, particularly if your anxiety is serious enough to impact large aspects of your life. Therapists are trained to help you deal with your problems and together, the two of you can begin fighting back your anxiety.

130.   Think about seeing a therapist or a psychologist. If your anxiety is based on stress that is affecting you in your life, it's a good idea to see someone who is an expert in dealing with these issues. There are many professionals who specialize in anxiety and know specific steps that you can take to feel better.

131.   Start writing in a gratitude journal. At the end of each day, write down at least five things you were grateful for. Become aware of all the wonderful positive things in your life and shift your focus away from dwelling on things that trigger worry, stress or negativity.

132.   Coffee is a drink that you should try to avoid or limit at all costs in the morning and night. If you require energy, eat a piece of fruit instead of consuming coffee. Coffee contains a lot of caffeine and the heat from this drink can raise your anxiety level.

133.   Get more than one medical opinion. Different doctors treat different conditions differently. One doctor may prescribe anxiety medicine, while another might only recommend therapy. Get more than one opinion about what you can do so that you can conquer your anxiety, and make sure you understand all the options available to you.

134.   A good way to lessen anxiety is by paying your bills on time. Late payments may increase the amount of stress you feel and add to your anxiety. Keep up to date with paying your bills and you should notice a difference in your stress and anxiety.

135.   To help you cope with anxiety, stop thinking about future events that haven't occurred yet. When you think about something that hasn't happened, there is no way for you to know how it will turn out. Oftentimes, people will think negatively when they look into the future, and this causes unnecessary worry. So either only deal with the present, or change your thoughts about the future to more positive ones.

136.   Keeping yourself busy can really help reduce anxiety. Sometimes, simple tasks, such as, washing the dishes or raking the yard, will help

you stay busy. Most people have more than enough to do, so get excited about just a few projects that will keep you smiling.

137.   Choose a calming mantra that you can repeat to yourself when you feel anxious. Short, simple phrases work best, although some people prefer to chant a soothing sound. Select a mantra that is personally meaningful and that you can recall quickly. Repeat the mantra as often as needed, either in your head or out loud, if you are alone.

138.   If anxiety has taken over your life, get professional help. Nobody should have to suffer silently through the fear, or be forced to live a limited life due to anxiety. There is help available, so talk to a professional, or look online for a forum where you can discuss common issues with others. Doing nothing is condemning yourself to a miserable existence.

139.   Keep yourself as busy as possible at all times. When you have down time, it will be easier for your mind to focus on negative things and will, therefore, fuel anxiety. Start your day out by cleaning the house, working in the garden, reading a book or doing some other activity that you enjoy.

140.   If you have been prescribed medication for anxiety, be sure that you take it at the same time every day. You can put your bottle by your toothbrush in the cabinet, or just wherever you will notice it. Remember that some medications take a while to work, so you have to take it every day.

141.   If you often find yourself feeling anxious, stay busy. If you are just lounging around all day unoccupied, your mind will start to wander and begin thinking negative thoughts, causing you to feel anxious. Things that are simple, like cleaning your home or washing the car can help a lot.

142.   Try creating your own anxious worrying period. Choose a single or two 10 minute spots each day where you can worry and just feel anxious. During this worry period, try focusing only on the anxious, negative thoughts without trying to correct them. The rest of the day should remain anxiety-free.

143.   Avoid thinking about things that worry you by doing something else. Keep busy by gardening or even, reading a book. As soon as you wake up, start your day doing something to keep your mind free of anxiety. This will keep

your mind off of those things that bother you and cause you anxiety.

144.   Exercise is a great way to eliminate anxiety from your life. This is not only good for your body, but it is good for your mind, as well. Make sure that you do not overexert yourself, but take the time every day to get out and get active, in order to reduce your anxiety.

145.   It might seem funny, but silly things, like dancing around the house, can be a beneficial distraction. If you can laugh and relax, then you can stop anxiety from growing. Do whatever is needed in order to get out of this predicament.

146.   A great way to help you deal with your anxiety is to identify the things that bring it on. When you determine what causes your anxiety, you can better prepare yourself to deal with those situations should they arise in the future. This way, you can see what specific things you need to work on.

147.   Talk with friends and family about your anxiety. One of the best ways to get rid of it, is to let people know what you're feeling. When you talk to people about your life, your mood picks up and this makes you feel less anxious, in

general. You will get support from trusted friends and family and this helps in your battle against anxiety.

148.   Learning how to deal with stress is the key to reducing anxiety. Many people experience something known as floating anxiety because they are unaware of where the stress is actually coming from. This can be dealt with by finding the source of stress through professional therapy or other similar methods.

149.   Think about seeing a therapist or a psychologist. If your anxiety is based on stress that is affecting you in your life, it's a good idea to see someone who is an expert in dealing with these issues. There are many professionals who specialize in anxiety and know specific steps that you can take to feel better.

150.   You should always take time for your own interests if you are someone who suffers from anxiety. Working constantly or thinking about negative things can make your anxiety increase. All you need is one hour a day to read a book, watch tv or even take a nap.

151.   Deep breathing exercises can help more than almost anything to help diffuse feelings of

anxiety. Learning a few exercises will give you something helpful to do when you start feeling overwhelmed. It can be helpful to just breathe for a few minutes and then, you will feel calm enough to go on.

152.   Anxiety is not necessarily a bad thing, but when stress gets overwhelming, it causes physical and emotional problems. You need to focus on controlling the amount of anxiety in your life. It also helps to limit stressful anxiety and only acknowledge anxiety that motivates you.

153.   If you do not put some type of positive interaction in between you and your anxiety, it will continue to grow. No matter what you decide to do, when an anxiety attack occurs, try remaining positive about everything that goes through your mind. When something negative occurs, turn it into something positive.

154.   Meditate in the morning. Every morning, take fifteen minutes for yourself. Find a comfortable chair and close your eyes. Try to concentrate on a relaxing image, such as a peaceful scene, or the face of a loved one. If intrusive thoughts start to enter your head, repeat a mantra over and over, such as "I am relaxed".

155.   One of the ways that you can feel better during the day and help reduce anxiety is to stretch the moment that you wake up. This can help limit any strain on your body when you go to work or school and can help generate the relaxation of all your muscles.

156.   Consider your diet when dealing with anxiety. A diet that is high is sugar and unrefined carbohydrates can contribute to feelings of anxiety. It takes place because when you eat sugary foods, your blood sugar raises first. Then, you experience a blood sugar drop that can leave you feeling weak, anxious and craving more sugar, which only exacerbates the problem.

157.   For most people, anxiety is caused by worrying about things that haven't occurred yet. People often believe something negative will happen before anything even occurs. To help change this, you should not worry about things that may or may not happen in the future. If you think only bad things will happen in the future, then that is what you will get, which will only worsen your anxiety.

158.   Make an effort to find someone that you trust to talk about your worries with. If you're

dealing with anxiety, it's crucial that you find a strong support system. A friend might be able to help you find solutions and talking about your problems will make you feel much better.

159.   Avoid people that only bring you down. For instance, if someone you know always has something negative to say, you probably should avoid him or her as often as you can. These type of people are more likely to cause you stress and increase your anxiety.

160.   Learn to feel the anxiety in your body. Focus on where it is located, such as a tight chest feeling, and stay focused on it until the feeling dissolves. This may seem difficult at first, but with just a bit of practice you will be able to release anxious feelings within seconds or a few minutes.

161.   If you continually experience high levels of stress, even after trying to deal with it in other ways, exercise can be a great idea. It helps to reduce stress naturally, by allowing you to work through stressful situations, but also by releasing different hormones that can actually minimize stress levels.

162.   Eat a better diet. The foods you eat might have a lot to do with the anxiety you are dealing with on a daily basis. Super foods containing a lot of vitamins and minerals might be the key to ridding yourself from the anxiety you are battling in your life.

163.   It can be difficult to escape the stress of life in the fast lane, but you can reduce your anxiety by organizing the obligations in your life according to importance. Prioritize events and eliminate anything which really is not necessary. Free up enough time so you can relax several times each week.

164.   What is causing your anxiety? Can you find a way to face these fears? Confronting and dealing with the source of your anxiety will take time and effort, but in the end it is better than avoiding it for the rest of your life. The therapeutic benefits of realizing that you can overcome anxiety will propel you into more changes in the future.

165.   Keep tabs on or eliminate your consumption of caffeine, nicotine and other stimulants. These substances increase your heart rate and can make you feel more jittery and anxious than you already do. If you cannot make it through the day without several cups of java, look at the

reasons why and find ways to make your day less hectic.

166.   When you wake up in the morning, take a multivitamin to help reduce your stress level as the day wears on. Multivitamins contain a lot of valuable nutrients that can help to create a balance in your body and transport the necessary minerals to the areas that need it the most.

167.   A good way to get rid of your anxiety is to treat yourself to a snack that you like. When you start to feel a bit anxious, one of the best ways to calm yourself, is to make your taste buds happy. When you make your taste buds happy, your stomach is happy, and then you're happy.

168.   Do not worry alone. When your worrisome thoughts go unchecked, they can easily spiral into terrible doomsday scenarios unnecessarily. Call a friend or supportive loved one, and run your fears past them. They can probably offer you some reassurance and perspective on what is bothering you, keeping your fears under control.

169.   Keep yourself as busy as possible at all times. When you have down time, it will be easier for your mind to focus on negative things and will, therefore, fuel anxiety. Start your day out by

cleaning the house, working in the garden, reading a book or doing some other activity that you enjoy.

170. Try to have a thicker skin when you are dealing with your emotions. If you have strong feelings about something, you are more likely to feel negative about something and worry, which leads to serious anxiety issues. Practice some emotional detachment when you are going through your everyday proceedings.

171. If anxiety and concern seems to overwhelm every waking moment, consider setting aside a specific time in which you allow yourself to think about the things that worry you the most. By restricting your worrying time to this period only, you will be able to free-up the rest of your day to focus on positive, productive aspects of life.

172. Relieve your unfounded worries, by doing some research. Statistics, facts, and other pieces of information can help you feel more secure. Learning more about what is bothering you can also show you that you don't, in fact, have anything to worry about. If doing the research yourself might worsen your anxiety, ask a friend, or family member to help.

173.	Breathing techniques are one of the best ways that you can reduce all physical stress that causes anxiety as the day wears on. Take long, deep breaths during the day to let your body acquire the oxygen that it needs to function properly. Engaging in this breathing pattern helps stabilize mood and reduces tension.

174.	Cut your intake of nicotine and alcohol. Many people think these substances relax you, but in reality they don't. In fact, using these substances can lead to a lot more anxiety than was there to begin with. Instead, seek natural relaxation alternatives, get out more, and watch what you are eating.

175.	Set aside a specific time to focus on your worries and doubts. Tell yourself that you cannot worry all day, and that you have to wait until the scheduled time to worry. Give yourself an hour to address your problems. When you are finished with this time out, do not let yourself focus on these issues. This approach is a wonderful, structured way to control the mind.

176.	Learn to accept your failings. You are not a superhero. You cannot save the world, nor does the world expect that of you. You may feel that your personal issues are world-altering; however, the reality is, they are simply obstacles to overcome. Realize that you are not expected to be perfect and have all the answers; you are only human.

177.   Start writing in a gratitude journal. At the end of each day, write down at least five things you were grateful for. Become aware of all the wonderful positive things in your life and shift your focus away from dwelling on things that trigger worry, stress or negativity.

178.   Seek good association. It is very important to remain social, in order to, stay happy and as worry free as possible. Not only that, but without someone providing feedback to you, it is very common for people to create worst case scenarios in their head about the anxieties they are dealing with.

179.   Listen to music. However, not just any music will do. The next time you feel your anxiety levels rising, throw on your favorite CD, or playlist. Whether you enjoy the calming sounds of a classical orchestra, or rocking out to 80's hair metal, you will feel your anxiety melt away with each song you know by heart. Before you know it, the anxiety is reduced, if not gone, and your spirits will be invigorated and renewed.

180.   Give it time. Sometimes the healing process from anxiety related issues can be very gradual. Many times you might not feel like you are making any progress at all. The key to this is to understand that it takes time. When you look back over the months you will notice your progress, and after a year, you will be able to notice a significant change.

181.   Learn how to distract yourself. As soon as you feel the anxiety starting to overwhelm you, find something that offers a distraction. Make sure that it's something that takes up a lot of concentration or energy, such as a difficult puzzle or a brisk workout. By concentrating on something other than your anxiety, you will find that it disappears quite quickly.

182.   When anxiety is getting the better of you, get some exercise. Exercise boosts levels of brain chemicals like serotonin, and dopamine, which help you feel happier and more relaxed. Physical activity can also be a great stress-reliever, and reducing your stress can certainly have positive impacts on your anxiety levels.

183.   Keeping yourself busy can really help reduce anxiety. Sometimes, simple tasks, such as,

washing the dishes or raking the yard, will help you stay busy. Most people have more than enough to do, so get excited about just a few projects that will keep you smiling.

184.   Learn how to have control over your feelings and do not let them get the best of you. If you allow your feelings to take over in everyday situations it will only lead to more anxiety. Take a few deep breaths and think things through before letting things get out of control.

185.   Self discipline is a great way to get a hold of your emotions. If you can control your emotions, then you can control your anxiety. Your anxiety attacks are fueled by negative feelings. Being mindful of your emotions and viewing emotions as passing feelings, rather than the true essence of yourself, will help you to gain control.

186.   To compensate for a tendency to breathe too fast during an anxious period, practice deep breathing exercises routinely so they are second nature when you need them. Anxiety may cause you to hyperventilate. Force yourself to breathe deeply and from your diaphragm. Concentrate on pushing your stomach in and out to see that you breath deeply and keep your anxiety under control.

187.   When you are suffering from high anxiety and stress, your body may keep you awake, at times, and cause insomnia. There are a number of natural sleep aids on the market that can help you sleep, or you can go to the doctor and try using a prescription that can help you get the sleep your body needs.

188.   If your anxiety is so bad that you have a hard time sleeping you should adjust your nightly ritual accordingly. Avoid watching things like horror films and action movies that creates negative feelings that persist once you go to bed. Try watching more relaxing programming or listening to music before you head to bed.

189.   Making sure you get sufficient sleep is vital to successfully combating anxiety. Lack of sufficient sleep not only affects the physical body, but also the mind. This contributes to anxiety. Experts strongly recommend that adults get 7-8 hours each night of good quality sleep.

190.   You should try to add some deep breathing techniques to your daily schedule, if you are suffering from feelings of anxiety. If you breathe from the diaphragm, it brings oxygen to your blood and that will help you to relax right away.

Any time that you feel overwhelmed, you should take a minute to do this.

191.   Reduce the anxiety in your life by learning to say no to situations that cause you stress. There is no reason to feel that you must be available to fulfill every request that is asked of you. Learn not to accept responsibility for more than you are able to handle comfortably.

192.   Make it a habit of staying in the moment or focusing on today. You need to stop obsessing over past problems or future fears. This can cause panic, worry, and other emotions which causes panic attacks. Minimize anxiety by thinking only about your current activity.

193.   Volunteer in your community. Finding something that really makes you feel good about doing it, will have a very positive impact in your life. The happier you are, the less anxious you will feel. You could work at a homeless shelter, read to kids at the library, or work at an animal shelter. Whatever makes you feel the best will help you the most.

194.   If you feel like nothing is working for your anxiety and your doctor recommends it, take medication. Many people do not like the idea of

relying on medication for assistance, but sometimes, it is the only thing that works. But, only resort to this if your doctor feels it is needed.

195.   One way to cope with anxiety is to just breathe! By focusing on your breathing and taking slow, even breaths is one of the easiest ways to relax. Start by counting to five as you inhale, then exhale for the same amount of time. You'll start to feel calmer, and you'll buy yourself some time to deal with a difficult situation.

196.   When you are starting to let anxiety get on top of you, use visual anchors. This means when you are feeling anxiety creep in to your thoughts look up to the clouds, or try to find some water to look at to calm you down. You could even use a stress ball.

197.   Anxiety can take a lot out of you, both emotionally and physically. On top of seeing a physician, you should have an organized plan in place. Without organization, dealing with your anxiety will become sporadic and unhealthy. You must be organized when coping and dealing with your anxiety attacks.

198.   If you have an anxiety problem, then you should cut down on sugar and caffeine. Sometimes these things can make you feel even more nervous than usual. If you must have caffeine or sugar, then at least cut back. Your diet plays a crucial role in how you react to anxiety.

199.   Learn helpful techniques to help you through anxiety, be it, deep breathing, mental exercises or quiet music. Be aware of what will work for you when you feel overwhelmed by anxiety so that you are able to address it in some way. This will help you get through and give you some much needed control.

200.   Talk to a trusted friend or family member about your anxiety problems. If you tell someone else how you feel, they may be able to help you put things in perspective and help you to think positive thoughts. This can help you get rid of anxiety or at least make it better.

201.   Try to stay busy as much as you can when you are dealing with anxiety. While meditation and deep breathing exercises are a good idea, other things that keep you idle are not good for you. Staying active will keep your mind off of all

the things that are creating your feelings of anxiety.

202.   You can use exercise to get rid of anxiety. Exercise can help you keep busy and get healthy at the same time. It also keeps you from thinking negatively. Exercise is also known to release endorphins in your brain. These give you a natural high and help relieve tension that can cause anxiety.

203.   Learn to breathe deeply from your diaphragm. When you take deep, regular breaths from your diaphragm, you will increase your calming feelings and begin to relax. Focus on breathing from your midsection, near your belly button. The stomach should extend outwards, if the breath is coming from the right area.

204.   Avoid thinking about things that worry you by doing something else. Keep busy by gardening or even, reading a book. As soon as you wake up, start your day doing something to keep your mind free of anxiety. This will keep your mind off of those things that bother you and cause you anxiety.

205.   Learn to embrace the uncertain. Things happen that you cannot predict and there is

nothing you can do about it. Worrying does not help. Instead, you will find yourself unable to enjoy anything in life. Learn to accept the things that you cannot control and learn not to look for instant solutions when it comes to the problems you have in life.

206.   Work your anxiety out with exercise. Sometimes, anxiety is just a bunch of pent-up energy that needs to be worked off. Swim, bike, go to the gym or do some vigorous and energetic cleaning around the house. Channel anxious feelings into a project that you have been putting off, and use the anxious energy to get the work done.

207.   Boost your serotonin levels with a good workout! Low levels of serotonin are known to trigger feelings of anxiety, but exercising can fix this. Brisk walks with your dog, gym workouts and even gardening can all promote brain production of both dopamine and serotonin, which are natural relaxants. This not only helps with anxiety, but it helps with depression too.

208.   No one wants to admit that they have an issue with anxiety. It can be embarrassing to be sweaty, nervous, clammy, and jittery in front of other people. You can avoid this somewhat by

knowing what things make you so anxious and either working on facing your fears or avoiding situations that will bring them about.

209.   Have you been screened for depression? Many people who have anxiety disorders or just high levels of anxiety in general, are also depressed. This depression could be causing your anxiety, or could be caused by it, but either way, treating your depression will help you to feel better and manage your symptoms better.

210.   You should always take time for your own interests if you are someone who suffers from anxiety. You will not find relief from anxiety or stress if you don't take time out from daily pressures. Allocate yourself one single hour to do something that you love, whether it be reading, crafts or an episode of your favorite TV show.

211.   When excessive worry, and anxiety takes control of your mind, stop, and write down the things that are bothering you. Putting your worries in writing, allows you to see, and evaluate the source of your anxiety. Take action on the things that you can resolve. Release the items that are beyond your control.

212.   Anxiety can take a lot out of you, both emotionally and physically. On top of seeing a physician, you should have an organized plan in place. Without organization, dealing with your anxiety will become sporadic and unhealthy. You must be organized when coping and dealing with your anxiety attacks.

213.   A great tip to help reduce the amount of anxiety you feel is to cut back on your caffeine intake. Caffeine is a stimulant which only increases the anxiousness or nervousness you are already feeling. Reducing the amount of caffeine you take will help reduce the amount of anxiety you feel.

214.   Anxiety is often based on external, rather than internal, factors. Because of this,it is essential to pinpoint the causes of stress, and anxiety. Once these problem areas have been located, it is possible to attempt to remove them from your life. If you are unable to remove them completely, you can, perhaps, diminish them.

215.   To help you reduce your anxiety symptoms, keep a journal of all of the events or issues that make you anxious throughout the day. Refer back to these events and see how they actually transpired. You will realize that you are often

imagining a worst case scenario which does not transpire.

216. One way to deal with anxiety is with music. If you are experiencing anxiety, go ahead and listen to your favorite album. Focus on each note in the music. Soon, you will be able to forget the things that are making you anxious. Keeping your mind focused on something else goes a long way toward relieving anxiety.

217. If worldly issues cause you to feel anxious, limit your exposure to television and newspapers. Only give yourself enough time to keep up with essential current events, and avoid allowing yourself to be brought down by negative news topics.

218. Consider your diet when dealing with anxiety. A diet that is high is sugar and unrefined carbohydrates can contribute to feelings of anxiety. It takes place because when you eat sugary foods, your blood sugar raises first. Then, you experience a blood sugar drop that can leave you feeling weak, anxious and craving more sugar, which only exacerbates the problem.

219. When you are on anxiety medication, never stop taking it without talking to your doctor.

Even if you feel like you are better, you still cannot just stop. Some of these medications can make you very ill and can even be deadly if you just stop all of a sudden.

220.   Watch how much alcohol you drink. If you are going out with your friends to drink, then try to reduce your alcohol consumption. Alcohol can do damage to your body while increasing the amount of stress that you have in the long-term. Also, alcohol puts you in many dangerous situations that can yield more anxiety.

221.   Don't forget to play. With the hustle and bustle of your busy life, taking the time to play a sport, a game or an instrument might seem frivolous. Taking an hour to let your hair down and have fun can do wonders for your stress and anxiety levels, though.

222.   Remaining sedentary and focusing on the negative is not likely to help things. Instead, look for ways to become busy that you could keep your mind out of your worries. Find something you enjoy, which is keep your mind busy, and decrease anxiety.

223.   Make sure that you are not alone in your room for long periods of time. One of the best

things that you can do is to go out with friends and share time with the people that you love. This can help you to reduce anxiety and inject fun into your day.

224.   If anxiety and concern seems to overwhelm every waking moment, consider setting aside a specific time in which you allow yourself to think about the things that worry you the most. By restricting your worrying time to this period only, you will be able to free-up the rest of your day to focus on positive, productive aspects of life.

225.   Make time for practicing some relaxation techniques. There are various techniques that you can work into your schedule too. Relaxation techniques like progressive muscle relaxation, mindfulness meditation, and some deep breathing may reduce your anxiety symptoms, and help you feel more relaxed so you can have a better emotional well-being.

226.   After being diagnosed with anxiety disorder, many people worry about the cost associated with needed medical intervention. Most insurance plans will cover needed medicines and treatments for this disorder. If you currently do not have health insurance, contact your county government's Health and Human Services

division. In many instances, they offer mental health care at a nearby public health facility. Charges at these facilities are pro-rated on a person's ability to pay.

227.   Use deep breathing techniques to calm anxiety. Try to breathe in for six counts and then out for six counts, through the nose. This will relax the central nervous system and calm anxious feelings. Since breathing can be done anywhere, this is a great on-the-spot treatment for anxiety.

228.   A lot of people enjoy a nice cup of hot tea to offset anxiety. This could be a good relaxation technique, but do not neglect having medical advice. If your anxiety does not decrease after a length of time, it is important to follow up with a doctor if you are ever to get better.

229.   Be aware that you don't have to face anxiety alone. Just look at the huge selection of supplements in your local health food store, and you can see that there are literally millions of people who suffer from anxiety. Keep this in mind when you are feeling isolated, there are others out there and you can find help.

230.	Anxiety is often based on external, rather than internal, factors. Because of this,it is essential to pinpoint the causes of stress, and anxiety. Once these problem areas have been located, it is possible to attempt to remove them from your life. If you are unable to remove them completely, you can, perhaps, diminish them.

231.	If anxiety is getting the best of you, consider joining a support group or online forum. It really helps to talk with others who are going through the same thing that you are feeling and they can often offer you ways of coping you may not have thought of before. It can also be a great way to meet people you can relate to, and vice-versa.

232.	There is no magic bullet to treat anxiety, it has to be treated in a professional manner by professionals. If you have seen advertisements for medications or miracle cures, do not believe them. Many times the treatment of anxiety can only be achieved over time, so do not believe in the snake charmers.

233.	If you are experiencing anxiety at work, which seems to be making it hard to get your job done, it may help to see a therapist. The therapist may help you to find out what it is that is causing you distress. It may be a co-worker, too much work to get done, or other job-related problems that can be easily fixed.

234.   Find a hobby. When your mind is idle, it is free to worry. Instead of sitting and dwelling on whatever is making you anxious, find something that you enjoy doing to serve as a distraction. If you don't have a hobby already, start looking for one. Whether you start knitting, constructing model cars, or restoring old furniture, you give your mind something to focus on besides the fear. As a bonus, having a hobby that you enjoy can reduce your stress levels all around.

235.   Many of those who have been professionally diagnosed as having an anxiety disorder will receive great benefit from joining and being active in a support or self-help group. Within the group, your day-to-day problems, plus personal achievements, can be shared with those who understand best, the ramifications of this disorder.

236.   Establish a goal for each day, and stay focused on achieving it. You will be able to focus on what is important and feel good about yourself, reducing the feeling that you have lost control of your anxiety. Try putting your thoughts into positive, constructive ideas.

237.   Anxiety can be caused by many different factors, so it is important to understand the root causes before trying to treat them. If you are unable to pinpoint exactly why you are feeling anxious, you will be unable to learn how to remove this anxiety in an easy and quick method.

238.   Try staying active. Exercise is a great way to let out some of your tensions and worries that have been plaguing you. It can put any negative thoughts far away from you and it naturally creates positive thoughts for you to dwell on, instead! Make sure that you go to the gym!

239.   Try to develop healthier eating habits. Begin your day the right way by eating some breakfast, then keep going with small, frequent meals throughout your day. Going without eating for too long during the day can cause your blood sugar to lower, which can make you feel much more anxious.

240.   Reduce your level of anxiety by asking others for help when you need it. Many people feel that asking for help is a sign of weakness, but it is actually a very intelligent thing to do when a task is more than you can handle. Delegating

appropriate tasks to others will keep anxiety under control.

241.   Write a letter to your greatest fear about why you are so worried about it. Be sure to write exactly why it is making you feel that way and how it is affecting you. Now write a hate letter to your greatest anxiety, then battle it through the letter and dismiss it!

242.   Learning how to deal with stress is the key to reducing anxiety. Many people experience something known as floating anxiety because they are unaware of where the stress is actually coming from. This can be dealt with by finding the source of stress through professional therapy or other similar methods.

243.   If you continually experience high levels of stress, even after trying to deal with it in other ways, exercise can be a great idea. It helps to reduce stress naturally, by allowing you to work through stressful situations, but also by releasing different hormones that can actually minimize stress levels.

244.   When excessive worry, and anxiety takes control of your mind, stop, and write down the things that are bothering you. Putting your

worries in writing, allows you to see, and evaluate the source of your anxiety. Take action on the things that you can resolve. Release the items that are beyond your control.

245.   Some great supplements to take if you are experiencing anxiety are cod liver, krill or fish oil. There have been studies that have shown that these three oils are as effective as many of the prescription medications that are available on the market for treating anxiety and depression. A good rule of thumb is 1,000 to 2,000 mg, per day.

246.   Stay away from people that make you nervous. That advice probably sounds obvious, but many anxiety sufferers take on discomforts for fear of upsetting others. Being around people who make you uncomfortable will cause you unnecessary stress and worsen your anxiety.

247.   There are many herbs that you can research, if you want to control your anxiety. Some of them include passionflower, chamomile, kava kava, and St. John's Wort. However, prior to taking anything for your anxiety, including herbal remedies, it is important that you consult with a medical professional.

248.   You may need to see a doctor because anxiety can be too much to deal with on your own. You may want to consider seeking assistance from a professional. If at all possible, visit a doctor who is already familiar with your medical history. He or she will be better equipped to advise you about what to do next.

249.   Separate yourself from things that cause you anxiety for a few hours every day. If you find that thinking about something too often is making you anxious, go on a walk or somewhere you like for a while. Thinking about something too much can just make it worse, so keep your mind occupied.

250.   Breathe easy. When you start to feel anxious, try to concentrate on breathing correctly. Inhale through your nostrils for about two seconds, and then exhale through parted lips for four seconds. Continue this routine for a full minute. Once your breathing gets back to normal, follow it up with a couple of minutes of soothing, positive self-talk.

251.   Social interaction is a must for people, in order to survive. You will die slowly without any social interaction. It is also a big help when it comes to dealing with anxiety. Try talking to

someone, and maybe, that person can help talk you through your anxiety by helping you sort things out.

252.	One of the ways that you can feel better during the day and help reduce anxiety is to stretch the moment that you wake up. This can help limit any strain on your body when you go to work or school and can help generate the relaxation of all your muscles.

253.	Find a trusted person. Discuss your anxiety with this person when you can. Having someone you trust to confide in can really make a big difference. Keeping your feelings bottled up inside makes things worse.

254.	Do not fear seeking medical advice for facing your anxiety. Just the thought of seeking a professional opinion, can be another source of anxiety. Don't let this happen to you. Anxiety is often a medical condition that can be solved with the right information and treatment. Relax and make the appointment.

255.	Find something else to focus on. Instead of thinking about whatever it is that is causing your anxiety, find something calm, peaceful and serene to focus on. It could be a good memory, a future dream or goal, or just something that you find calm and soothing. Don't forget to take deep breaths as you do this.

256.   Take time to list what stresses you out in life. You should put the things that you can change on one side, and the ones that you cannot on the other. Focus on trying to change the things that you can; try to stop worrying about those that you cannot.

257.   It is okay to cry if you are depressed, or anxious. If you feel like crying, then you need to express yourself, and let those emotions out. There is a reason our bodies are designed to have tears, and to cry. It is so, that these emotions do not get trapped inside us, and cause bigger problems.

258.   Reduce your intake of alcohol and nicotine. Many people think these substances relax you, but in reality they don't. Ultimately, though, the chemicals in alcohol and cigarettes can actually exacerbate your anxiety. Instead, shift towards something that is healthy, such as relaxation therapies, a diet that is healthy and positive social activities.

259.   Is there something you know of that works to effectively eliminate anxiety? Laughing and smiling are easy ways to combat feelings of anxiety. Search for many things to be thankful for and happy with. In the midst of an anxiety attack, think about something funny that will give you a good laugh.

260.   Set aside a specific time to focus on your worries and doubts. Rigidly tell yourself as the day goes by that you could not dwell on these things before the allotted time. Make an hour available for addressing these things. Once you reach your time limit, put your mental focus elsewhere, and do not allow yourself to continue worrying. Scheduling in this way can be a very effective means of controlling anxiety in your life.

261.   A great way to help reduce the anxiety that you feel, is to take a ride with your friends to the spa. Soaking your body in a jacuzzi, or bath is a great way to relax, and put things in perspective. Also, the heat helps to you to sweat, and flush out the extra toxins in your body.

262.   Talk with friends and family about your anxiety. One of the best ways to get rid of it, is to let people know what you're feeling. When

you talk to people about your life, your mood picks up and this makes you feel less anxious, in general. You will get support from trusted friends and family and this helps in your battle against anxiety.

263.   If you continually experience high levels of stress, even after trying to deal with it in other ways, exercise can be a great idea. It helps to reduce stress naturally, by allowing you to work through stressful situations, but also by releasing different hormones that can actually minimize stress levels.

264.   Green tea is a great nutrient that you can add to your daily routine to help your anxiety level. Instead of drinking soda or fruit drinks, switch to green tea to help flush out the free radicals in your body and to create a soothing feeling, as soon as you consume it.

265.   Exercising on a regular basis is one way to deal with anxiety. Exercise is great for your anxiety because it is a natural "stress buster" that can relieve your anxiety symptoms. Try to get in a good half an hour workout to help relieve stress and feel better faster.

266.   If you are wanting to learn how to control your anxiety, you must have the ability to control your thoughts. Not having control over any of your thoughts, just makes your anxiety even worse. Having bad thoughts can lead to a panic attack really fast. If you start experiencing out-of-control thoughts, immediately stop what you are doing and take control.

267.   Dealing with anxiety before it paralyzes your actions is the best way to handle these feelings. If each situation is resolved with as it arises, the stress can be released and an anxiety attack can be avoided. Think calmly about the situation and decide on the best course of action.

268.   To help manage your anxiety, consider meeting with a therapist who specializes in cognitive behavioral therapy. This kind of therapy can help you attack specific fears or worries by identifying and changing distorted patterns in your thinking. By looking at the full picture of how your worries affect you, you can hopefully decrease your overall anxiety when those thinking patterns are eliminated.

269.   If you have an anxiety disorder, it may be wise to seek out a support group for people with anxiety disorder and panic attack. Being around

others who share your symptoms can be a great comfort and will allow you to share ideas for controlling anxiety and overcoming your fears.

270.   If you are suffering from anxiety, one of the best things that you can do is to drink a lot of water during the day. Eight glasses of water can help to reduce the toxins in your body and put you in the best position to stay positive during the day.

271.   Keep tabs on or eliminate your consumption of caffeine, nicotine and other stimulants. These substances increase your heart rate and can make you feel more jittery and anxious than you already do. If you cannot make it through the day without several cups of java, look at the reasons why and find ways to make your day less hectic.

272.   One of the ways that you can feel better during the day and help reduce anxiety is to stretch the moment that you wake up. This can help limit any strain on your body when you go to work or school and can help generate the relaxation of all your muscles.

273.   Talk to a trusted friend or family member about your anxiety problems. If you tell someone

else how you feel, they may be able to help you put things in perspective and help you to think positive thoughts. This can help you get rid of anxiety or at least make it better.

274.   Workplace anxiety can often be reduced or eliminated by taking a simple walk. As deadlines approach and employers pile on more work, many people forget the power of taking a short break. Going outside and walking around the building gives you a chance to refresh your mind and body.

275.   Speak with friends, family, or a doctor about your anxiety. You will only feel worse if you try to shell up all those bad thoughts and emotions. Giving mouth to those feelings can really enhance your mood and eliminate anxiety.

276.   Find a hobby. When your mind is idle, it is free to worry. Instead of sitting and dwelling on whatever is making you anxious, find something that you enjoy doing to serve as a distraction. If you don't have a hobby already, start looking for one. Whether you start knitting, constructing model cars, or restoring old furniture, you give your mind something to focus on besides the fear. As a bonus, having a hobby that you enjoy can reduce your stress levels all around.

277.   Many of those who have been professionally diagnosed as having an anxiety disorder will receive great benefit from joining and being active in a support or self-help group. Within the group, your day-to-day problems, plus personal achievements, can be shared with those who understand best, the ramifications of this disorder.

278.   Relieve your unfounded worries, by doing some research. Statistics, facts, and other pieces of information can help you feel more secure. Learning more about what is bothering you can also show you that you don't, in fact, have anything to worry about. If doing the research yourself might worsen your anxiety, ask a friend, or family member to help.

279.   Cut down on how much nicotine and alcohol you take in. Even though a lot of folks think that these two substances can induce relaxation, they don't. As a matter of fact, they can increase anxiety. Look for healthier and more positive ways to manage or reduce anxiety.

280.   Reward yourself, if you do things that have a positive impact on your life, in your work or someone else's life. Giving yourself the proper

acknowledgement for minor accomplishments will lead to greater success in your life. When you begin to see the positives about yourself, you begin to diminish the negatives.

281.	What does it take to eliminate anxiety from your life? Laughing and smiling are both things that can make anxiety a little less of a hassle. Stay conscious of the good things in your life. If you're having trouble and feel anxiety, laughing about things can really help. This can be a comedy show or maybe a funny song.

282.	Exercise is a great way to deal with your anxiety. Whenever you work out, you release a lot of tension or stress, which happens to be a major contributor to anxiety. When you get rid of this excess stress, you put yourself in a clearer state of mind, which should reduce the amount of anxiety you feel.

283.	Music can ease your anxiety. Playing an album you love can be a great idea when you feel anxiety coming on. Get into the music. Quite soon, your anxiety will be long forgotten. Keep your mind as busy as you can to deal with anxiety better.

284. Keep yourself as busy as you possibly can. Being very active helps prevent any anxiety that may occur. As soon as you get up in the mornings, begin doing something immediately. Make sure you keep yourself busy all day long. Clean up the house, walk the dog, clean up your garden, read, or exercise. All these things can decrease your anxiety. Remaining idle just causes you to think about the negative things that are occurring in your life, which makes your anxiety worse.

285. To compensate for a tendency to breathe too fast during an anxious period, practice deep breathing exercises routinely so they are second nature when you need them. When anxiety becomes especially intense, the tendency is to hyperventilate, breathing rapidly and shallowly. Instead, you should breathe deeply, from the diaphragm. You can lessen your anxiety by taking in full, deep breaths, and make sure your abdomen rises and falls.

286. Work on having good posture. Having bad posture compresses organs, cuts off circulation and shortens breathing. Many times, it is easy, even under a normal amount of anxiety, to sit in positions that cause harm to our body. Try not

to do this, as this will better your health and help decrease the amount of anxiety you endure.

287.   You should try to add some deep breathing techniques to your daily schedule, if you are suffering from feelings of anxiety. If you breathe from the diaphragm, it brings oxygen to your blood and that will help you to relax right away. Any time that you feel overwhelmed, you should take a minute to do this.

288.   Learn how to release anxious feelings with the help of emotional releasing techniques. Learn The Sedona Method or the Emotional Freedom Technique. These methods help you get to the root of your anxiety, and keep releasing it until you are completely relaxed. The information on these methods is either free or low-cost and can be found through a web search.

289.   Keep a log or a journal to try to figure out what your triggers are. Once you have the triggers mapped out, you will have a better idea of what you can do to reduce the anxiety that you feel in the different situations. Each situation may require a different management technique.

290.   Green tea is a great nutrient that you can add to your daily routine to help your anxiety level.

Instead of drinking soda or fruit drinks, switch to green tea to help flush out the free radicals in your body and to create a soothing feeling, as soon as you consume it.

291.   If anxiety is an issue, "me" time is very important. Too much hard work and not enough time to relax is a primary cause of anxiety and stress. Take some time to lay down, read a book or watch TV.

292.   Exercising regularly can benefit those who suffer with anxiety. Exercise is a great way to alleviate anxiety symptoms and can also get rid of stress. For results that work sooner rather than later, you should work out for half an hour almost every day.

293.   Do not watch television news. If you feel anxious as a result of hearing about robberies, car wrecks, murders and shootings, avoid exposing yourself to the news. On the whole, news tends to focus on the negative. They rarely have news reports about all of the positive things that take place every single day.

294.   Seek good association. It is very important to remain social, in order to, stay happy and as worry free as possible. Not only that, but without

someone providing feedback to you, it is very common for people to create worst case scenarios in their head about the anxieties they are dealing with.

295.   You aren't alone in your anxious struggles. Take a moment to look around you, and you'll realize that many people suffer with similar feelings of anxiety. Just remember, you aren't alone and there are ways you can treat anxiety.

296.   Try creating your own calming herbal tea tonic to help you with anxiety. There are many calming herbs out there that can help you deal with anxiety. Do your research and ask your doctor before combining any of them. You are bound to find one or two that can help you!

297.   Use exercise as a way to relieve your anxiety symptoms. No matter what it is, whether it's jogging around the block, biking, or swimming, getting your heart rate going is a great way to reduce anxiety. Research has shown that aerobic exercise is just as good as SSRIs at relieving mild to moderate anxiety. So get moving!

298.   Keep a journal for writing down any situation that produces feelings of anxiety. Over time, your journal will reveal patterns and

triggers for your anxiety episodes. It is then much easier to develop strategies for dealing with the triggers. You will be better able to avoid placing yourself in anxiety producing situations in the future.

299.   You may want to take fish oil, if you suffer from anxiety. Recent studies have shown that fish oil, not only helps prevent some physical ailments, but it helps with anxiety as well. But, prior to taking fish oil, speak with your doctor to make sure it is right for you.

300.   If you frequently suffer from bouts of anxiety that appear seemingly out of nowhere, or you feel anxious a majority of the time, you may have what is called generalized anxiety disorder. This disorder needs to be treated by an experienced doctor, or therapist before anxiety has a chance to take over your life.

301.   Try writing down what worries you. Carry a spare pad and pencil on you wherever you go, or type it on a smartphone, laptop, or tablet. When you are feeling anxious, try writing down what worries you. Writing it down is much harder than simply thinking about it, so the negative thoughts may disappear sooner.

302. If you find yourself feeling overly anxious, get outside and get some exercise. Exercise has many benefits for your whole body, and a good workout can really clear your mind and help improve your mood. You do not have to head to the gym or the pool, if you do not want to. Just taking a walk can help.

303. Avoid watching TV programs that cause you anxiety. For some people, watching the news can bring on an anxiety attack. Simply because there are many negative things the news covers. If it causes you stress, then turn it off, and watch something else that makes you happy, and anxiety free.

304. Always make it a point to focus on the positive things that are happening in your life, no matter how big or small it may be. Positive thoughts drown out the negative ones and the more positive thoughts you have, the smaller the problems in your life, will seem to you.

305. Make time for practicing some relaxation techniques. There are various techniques that you can work into your schedule too. Relaxation techniques like progressive muscle relaxation, mindfulness meditation, and some deep breathing may reduce your anxiety symptoms,

and help you feel more relaxed so you can have a better emotional well-being.

306.   Relieve your unfounded worries, by doing some research. Statistics, facts, and other pieces of information can help you feel more secure. Learning more about what is bothering you can also show you that you don't, in fact, have anything to worry about. If doing the research yourself might worsen your anxiety, ask a friend, or family member to help.

307.   Reduce your consumption of nicotine and alcohol. Many people think that these types of substances will relax you, but this is a mistake. In fact, they could lead to you experiencing more anxiety. Focus on healthier alternatives to stress reduction, such as social activities, relaxation techniques, and a nutritious diet.

308.   Schedule yourself a time of day when you can think about what worries you. Firmly remind yourself that you can only think about those topics during the specified period. Allot an hour to address these things. When you have reached the end of your scheduled time, go back to not allowing yourself to focus on them. This approach can help you form better control.

309. When you begin to feel overwhelmed, or anxious, give yourself a time-out. Do some yoga, play pleasant music, learn techniques to relax, or get a massage. Taking a step back, and regaining your composure should stop the attack in its tracks, before it turns into a full blown anxiety attack.

310. Talk with friends and family about your anxiety. One of the best ways to get rid of it, is to let people know what you're feeling. When you talk to people about your life, your mood picks up and this makes you feel less anxious, in general. You will get support from trusted friends and family and this helps in your battle against anxiety.

311. If you continually experience high levels of stress, even after trying to deal with it in other ways, exercise can be a great idea. It helps to reduce stress naturally, by allowing you to work through stressful situations, but also by releasing different hormones that can actually minimize stress levels.

312. If your anxiety level is at an all time high you can help your mood by engaging in some type of healthy sexual activity. When people have sex it releases endorphins into the blood, which will

send signals to the brain that it needs to be in a much better mood.

313.   Use deep breathing techniques to calm anxiety. Try to breathe in for six counts and then out for six counts, through the nose. This will relax the central nervous system and calm anxious feelings. Since breathing can be done anywhere, this is a great on-the-spot treatment for anxiety.

314.   Consider alternative remedies. There are a number of things you can do to deal with your anxiety that fall outside of mainstream medicine. Give acupuncture a try, or perhaps some nutritional supplements. If you do practice these methods, be absolutely sure to notify your doctor to make sure it is safe for you to do.

315.   If you enjoy animals and live in a place where you can have a pet, then get a dog or a cat. A daily walk, enjoying nature with your dog is very relaxing and the exercise will do you good. Also, nothing is more calming than hearing your cat purr with contentment, while enjoying your company.

316.   While there are many possible medications, pills, and teas that are available for people who

suffer with anxiety and stress, the best medication is completely natural. The absolute best thing you can do to deal with high levels of anxiety is to take up a sport or begin exercising.

317.   Have a trusted resource to call on, whenever you may be subject to an attack. Be it a relative or friend, you should have someone who is aware of your condition and can help talk you through an attack. Having to face one alone is very overwhelming, and you will work through them quicker if you have someone to help.

318.   Focus your attention on the place where the anxiety is stemming from. You may feel this physically, and concentrating on it can reduce or eliminate it completely. If your attention starts to stray, just refocus yourself back to the place that is causing you anxiety for several minutes.

319.   A good way to get rid of your anxiety is to treat yourself to a snack that you like. When you start to feel a bit anxious, one of the best ways to calm yourself, is to make your taste buds happy. When you make your taste buds happy, your stomach is happy, and then you're happy.

320.   Try not to watch the news often. Many times, the news is filled with all kinds of negative

stories, about occurrences in your town, and around the world. When dealing with anxiety, you do not need to feed the anxiety anymore negative issues to dwell on. Turn off the TV, pick up a lighthearted book to read instead.

321.   If you are dealing with anxiety issues, one way to help is to change the way you think. Too much negative thinking can lead to anxiety. Instead of thinking the worst will happen, try to change your thought process into something that is positive. With positive thinking, you will begin to feel better.

322.   Keep yourself as busy as you possibly can. Being very active helps prevent any anxiety that may occur. As soon as you get up in the mornings, begin doing something immediately. Make sure you keep yourself busy all day long. Clean up the house, walk the dog, clean up your garden, read, or exercise. All these things can decrease your anxiety. Remaining idle just causes you to think about the negative things that are occurring in your life, which makes your anxiety worse.

323.   Talk to a trusted friend or family member about your anxiety problems. If you tell someone else how you feel, they may be able to help you

put things in perspective and help you to think positive thoughts. This can help you get rid of anxiety or at least make it better.

324.   It may seem like alcohol helps with anxiety, but it really is the opposite. Even though when you have a few drinks you anxiety seems to vanish, when you become dependent on it you actually create more anxiety. This is because you have to find ways to get more, and eventually become more sick than you were.

325.   Make sure that you are not alone in your room for long periods of time. One of the best things that you can do is to go out with friends and share time with the people that you love. This can help you to reduce anxiety and inject fun into your day.

326.   Practice staying in the present. A big problem that is common to those who suffer from anxiety is that they focus on past issues or future problems. All this will create is stressful feelings of worry, and this can bring on an anxiety episode. Reduce your anxiety by focusing on what you're currently doing and suspending other thoughts.

327.   If you are constantly feeling anxious, take a day for a professional massage. This will help to loosen up all of the knots in your body, and help eliminate the extra tension that you feel. Staying healthy physically is one of the best ways that you can improve your mental state.

328.   A helpful tip that you should think about in your times of stress is to have some snacks that contain carbohydrates. Eating these types of snacks will help to release serotonin in your brain. This is a natural occurring chemical that will make you feel good once it is released.

329.   If you feel like nothing is working for your anxiety and your doctor recommends it, take medication. Many people do not like the idea of relying on medication for assistance, but sometimes, it is the only thing that works. But, only resort to this if your doctor feels it is needed.

330.   When you are starting to let anxiety get on top of you, use visual anchors. This means when you are feeling anxiety creep in to your thoughts look up to the clouds, or try to find some water to look at to calm you down. You could even use a stress ball.

331.   A lot of introverted people suffer with social anxiety. Find activities to enjoy by yourself and with others so that if you do want to socialize at times, you can relax by sharing an enjoyable activity together.

332.   Make sure that you do not skip meals because it could lead you off on a path toward feelings of anxiety. When you do not eat correctly it throws your blood sugar out of whack. This may lead to feelings of panic in some situations. Make sure that you eat regularly.

333.   Try to avoid foods and drinks that contain high amounts of sugar. Not only can too much sugar affect your blood sugar levels, but it can also leave you jittery and cause anxiety. There are many sugar-free versions of foods and drinks that are just as good as their sugared versions.